Copyr

Table of Contents

Chapter 1: Understanding the Circadian Rhythm and Its Impact on Health

Quote: "The sun is but a morning star." - Henry David Thoreau

The human body operates on a remarkable internal clock, known as the circadian rhythm. Just as the sun rises and sets, our bodies have a natural ebb and flow that influences various physiological processes. Throughout history, great thinkers and philosophers have recognized the significance of this rhythmic pattern and its impact on our overall well-being. Henry David Thoreau, the renowned transcendentalist writer, alludes to the sun as a symbol of the circadian rhythm, suggesting that it marks the beginning of our daily journey. In this chapter, we embark on a captivating exploration of the circadian rhythm, diving deep into its profound influence on our health and vitality.

What is the Circadian Rhythm?

The circadian rhythm is an innate, approximately 24-hour cycle that regulates essential bodily functions, including sleep-wake patterns, hormone production, body temperature, metabolism, and even cognitive performance. It is a finely orchestrated symphony of molecular and cellular processes that synchronize with external cues, primarily light and darkness, to maintain optimal physiological balance.

Ancient civilizations, such as the Egyptians and Greeks, observed patterns of diurnal behavior in plants and animals, recognizing the recurrence of daily cycles. However, it was not until the 20th century that scientists began to unravel the intricacies of the circadian rhythm. Pioneering research by individuals like Franz Halberg and Colin Pittendrigh paved the way for a deeper understanding of this internal timekeeping system.

1.2 Importance of the Circadian Rhythm for Optimal Health

The circadian rhythm is not merely a concept limited to sleep-wake cycles; it plays a vital role in virtually every aspect of our health. Proper alignment of the circadian rhythm is crucial for maintaining physical and mental well-being. Numerous studies have revealed that disruptions to the circadian rhythm, such as shift work, jet lag, or irregular sleep patterns, can have detrimental effects on our health.

Sleep, a cornerstone of the circadian rhythm, is essential for memory consolidation, immune function, emotional regulation, and overall cognitive performance. A synchronized circadian rhythm ensures that we experience restful and restorative sleep, waking up refreshed and energized for the day ahead.

Furthermore, the circadian rhythm influences hormone production, including melatonin, cortisol, insulin, and leptin, which are key players in metabolism, appetite regulation, and weight management. Disruptions to this delicate balance can contribute to metabolic disorders, obesity, and even chronic conditions like diabetes.

1.3 How Diet Affects the Circadian Rhythm

While light and darkness are the primary drivers of the circadian rhythm, emerging evidence suggests that our dietary choices can also influence its function. The field of chrononutrition explores the intricate relationship between food and the circadian rhythm, emphasizing that not only when we eat but also what we eat matters.

Certain nutrients and bioactive compounds found in foods can directly interact with the circadian clock genes, modulating their expression and activity. For instance, polyphenols in fruits and vegetables, such as resveratrol in grapes and quercetin in onions, have been shown to impact circadian gene expression and promote health.

Moreover, the timing of meals and the duration of fasting periods, referred to as time-restricted eating (TRE), can have a profound impact on circadian alignment. By aligning our eating patterns with our natural circadian rhythm, we can optimize metabolic function, promote weight management, and enhance overall health.

In the following chapters, we will delve deeper into the fascinating science behind the circadian rhythm, exploring its biological underpinnings, the influence of light and darkness, and practical strategies for implementing a circadian diet to maximize your well-being.

So, join us on this captivating journey as we unlock the secrets of the circadian rhythm and discover the profound impact it has on our health, vitality, and overall quality of life. As Thoreau reminds us, the sun may be just a morning star, but our circadian rhythm is the guiding light that shapes our daily existence.

Chapter 2: The Science behind the Circadian Diet

Quote: "Our task must be to free ourselves... by widening our circle of compassion to embrace all living creatures and the whole of nature and its beauty." - Albert Einstein

Albert Einstein, the brilliant physicist and philosopher, recognized the interconnectedness of all living beings and the intricate beauty of nature. In the realm of the circadian rhythm, this quote resonates profoundly as we delve into the scientific foundations of the circadian diet. In this chapter, we embark on a captivating exploration of the science behind the circadian rhythm, uncovering the intricate mechanisms that govern our internal clocks and how they intersect with nutrition and metabolism. By understanding this underlying science, we can unlock the keys to optimal health and well-being.

2.1 Circadian Biology and Metabolism:

The foundation of the circadian rhythm lies within our biology, particularly in the intricate web of molecular and cellular processes that govern our internal clocks. The master regulator of the circadian rhythm is the suprachiasmatic nucleus (SCN), a cluster of specialized cells located in the hypothalamus of the brain. The SCN receives input from light-sensitive cells in the eyes, relaying information about the presence or absence of light.

These light cues synchronize our internal clocks with the external environment, facilitating the harmonious functioning of various bodily systems. One of the key systems regulated by the circadian rhythm is metabolism. The circadian clock genes control the expression of genes involved in nutrient metabolism, energy balance, and the regulation of insulin sensitivity.

Research has shown that disruptions to the circadian rhythm, such as irregular sleep patterns or night-time eating, can lead to metabolic dysregulation, obesity, and an increased risk of chronic diseases. By understanding the intricate relationship between circadian biology and metabolism, we can harness the power of the circadian diet to optimize metabolic health and promote overall well-being.

2.2 Circadian Clock Genes and Their Role in Nutrition:

Deep within our cells, a set of genes known as clock genes intricately orchestrate the daily rhythms of our bodies. These genes produce proteins that interact in a feedback loop, creating a self-sustaining circadian clock within each cell. Two key clock genes are known as "Clock" and "BMAL1," which initiate the activation of other clock genes and drive the rhythmic expression of various metabolic genes.

The expression of clock genes can be influenced by external cues, including light, food, and physical activity. Notably, emerging research has revealed that nutrients and bioactive compounds present in our diet can directly impact the expression and activity of clock genes. For example, polyunsaturated fatty acids, such as omega-3 fatty acids found in fatty fish, have been shown to modulate clock gene expression and promote circadian alignment.

Understanding the interplay between clock genes and nutrition opens up exciting possibilities for tailoring our diets to optimize circadian health. By selecting nutrient-dense foods that support circadian gene expression, we can create a harmonious symphony within our cells and promote optimal metabolic function.

2.3 Influence of Light and Dark Cycles on the Circadian Rhythm:

Light and darkness serve as the primary external cues that entrain our circadian rhythm. The presence of light, particularly blue light, suppresses the release of melatonin, a hormone that signals our body to prepare for sleep. In contrast, darkness promotes melatonin production, signaling the body to enter the restful state of sleep.

In our modern world, we are exposed to artificial light sources, such as electronic devices and indoor lighting, which can disrupt our natural light-dark cycles. Prolonged exposure to artificial light, especially during the evening and night hours, can interfere with melatonin production, leading to difficulties falling asleep and a disrupted circadian rhythm.

Additionally, exposure to natural sunlight during the day is crucial for maintaining a robust circadian rhythm. Sunlight exposure in the morning helps synchronize the internal clocks, promoting alertness and vitality throughout the day. By incorporating light management strategies, such as limiting exposure to artificial light in the evening and ensuring sufficient exposure to natural light during the day, we can optimize our circadian rhythm and support overall well-being.

2.4 Effects of Disrupted Circadian Rhythm on Health: Disruptions to the circadian rhythm can have far-reaching consequences for our health. Shift work, for instance, forces individuals to work during the night and sleep during the day, throwing their circadian clocks out of sync with their environment. This misalignment has been associated with an increased risk of various health conditions, including cardiovascular disease, metabolic disorders, gastrointestinal disturbances, and mood disorders.

Furthermore, social jet lag, a phenomenon characterized by significant discrepancies in sleep and wake times between workdays and free days, can also disrupt the circadian rhythm. This irregular sleep pattern, akin to experiencing jet lag without traveling, has been linked to an increased risk of obesity, insulin resistance, and poorer overall health.

Understanding the detrimental effects of circadian disruptions empowers us to take proactive steps to realign our internal clocks and mitigate the risks associated with a disrupted circadian rhythm. Through the implementation of a circadian diet and lifestyle strategies, we can restore balance and promote optimal health.

In the following chapters, we will delve deeper into the practical aspects of the circadian diet, exploring the core principles, meal timing strategies, and nourishing food choices that can help us synchronize our internal clocks and optimize our health and well-being.

Join us as we unravel the intricate science behind the circadian rhythm and discover how nutrition and lifestyle choices can unlock the power of our internal clocks. As Einstein reminds us, by widening our circle of compassion to embrace all living creatures, we can extend that compassion to ourselves by nurturing our bodies and aligning with the rhythm of nature.

Chapter 3: Getting Started with the Circadian Diet

Introduction: Embarking on a journey towards embracing the circadian diet is a transformative step towards optimizing your health and well-being. In this chapter, we dive deep into the practical aspects of getting started with the circadian diet. From assessing your current eating patterns to creating a personalized circadian diet plan, we will guide you through the process of implementing this lifestyle change successfully. So, fasten your seatbelts and get ready to embark on an exciting adventure towards better health and vitality.

3.1 Assessing Your Current Eating Patterns:

Before embarking on any dietary change, it's essential to assess your current eating patterns to understand how they align with the principles of the circadian diet. Take a moment to reflect on your daily routine and habits, considering factors such as meal timing, food choices, and portion sizes.

Consider keeping a food journal for a few days, documenting everything you eat and noting the times at which you consume your meals and snacks. This will provide valuable insights into your current eating patterns and potential areas for improvement.

Reflect on how closely your current routine aligns with the principles of the circadian diet. Are you consuming meals at regular intervals? Do you often indulge in late-night snacking? Are your food choices predominantly whole and nutrient-dense? By honestly assessing your eating habits, you can identify areas where adjustments may be necessary to optimize your circadian health.

3.2 Identifying Your Natural Eating Window:

One of the key principles of the circadian diet is aligning your eating window with your body's natural rhythms. Each individual has a unique chronotype, which refers to their genetically predetermined preference for being a "morning person" or an "evening person." Understanding your chronotype can help you identify your natural eating window, during which your body is primed for optimal digestion and nutrient absorption.

To determine your chronotype and natural eating window, consider factors such as your energy levels throughout the day, your preferences for morning or evening activities, and when you naturally feel hungry. Some individuals may thrive with an earlier eating window, starting their day with a nourishing breakfast and concluding their meals by early evening. Others may find their energy peaks later in the day, and they prefer a slightly delayed eating window.

By identifying your natural eating window, you can structure your meals and snacks to align with your body's internal rhythms, promoting optimal digestion and metabolic function.

3.3 Creating a Circadian Diet Plan:

Now that you have assessed your current eating patterns and identified your natural eating window, it's time to create a personalized circadian diet plan. This plan will serve as a roadmap, guiding you towards nourishing food choices, appropriate meal timings, and a balanced macronutrient distribution.

Start by incorporating whole, nutrient-dense foods into your diet. Focus on fresh fruits and vegetables, lean proteins, healthy fats, and whole grains. These foods provide a wealth of vitamins, minerals, antioxidants, and fiber that support overall health and vitality.

Consider incorporating time-restricted eating (TRE) into your plan, which involves condensing your daily eating window to a specific time frame. This can be an effective strategy for aligning your meals with your natural circadian rhythm. Experiment with different eating windows and meal timings to find what works best for you.

Pay attention to the balance of macronutrients in your meals. Aim to include a combination of proteins, carbohydrates, and fats in each meal to promote sustained energy levels and satiety. Opt for lean protein sources such as poultry, fish, tofu, or legumes, complex carbohydrates like whole grains and starchy vegetables, and healthy fats from sources like avocados, nuts, and olive oil.

Don't forget to stay hydrated throughout the day. Water plays a vital role in maintaining optimal bodily functions, so ensure you drink enough water to support your overall well-being.

3.4 Incorporating Circadian Lifestyle Practices:

The circadian diet goes beyond just meal timing and food choices. It encompasses a holistic approach to aligning with the natural rhythms of life. Consider incorporating circadian lifestyle practices that support your circadian health and enhance your overall well-being.

Prioritize quality sleep by establishing a consistent sleep routine and creating a sleep-friendly environment. Ensure your bedroom is cool, dark, and free from electronic devices that emit blue light, which can disrupt your natural sleep-wake cycle.

Engage in regular physical activity to support circadian alignment. Moderate exercise during the day promotes alertness and vitality, while avoiding intense exercise close to bedtime, which can interfere with sleep quality.

Spend time outdoors, particularly in the morning, to expose yourself to natural light. Natural light exposure helps regulate your internal clocks and promotes a sense of well-being.

Practice stress management techniques, such as meditation, deep breathing exercises, or engaging in activities that bring you joy and relaxation. Chronic stress can disrupt your circadian rhythm, so it's essential to find healthy ways to manage and reduce stress levels.

By incorporating these circadian lifestyle practices alongside your circadian diet, you create a synergistic approach that optimizes your overall health and well-being.

Conclusion: Congratulations! You have taken the first steps towards implementing the circadian diet into your life. By assessing your current eating patterns, identifying your natural eating window, and creating a personalized circadian diet plan, you are well on your way to optimizing your health and vitality.

Remember, the circadian diet is not a rigid set of rules but a flexible framework that adapts to your unique needs and preferences. Be open to experimentation and adjust your plan as necessary to find what works best for you.

In the next chapter, we will explore specific meal ideas and recipes that align with the principles of the circadian diet. So get ready to tantalize your taste buds with nourishing and delicious culinary creations that support your circadian health and leave you feeling energized and satisfied.

Chapter 4: Nourishing Meal Ideas and Recipes for the Circadian Diet

Welcome to the culinary exploration of the circadian diet! In this chapter, we will dive into a world of nourishing meal ideas and recipes that align with the principles of the circadian diet. Prepare to tantalize your taste buds with exciting flavors, nutrient-dense ingredients, and innovative culinary creations. From breakfast to dinner, and everything in between, we have curated a collection of recipes that will inspire and delight you on your circadian journey.

4.1 Energizing Breakfast Options:

They say breakfast is the most important meal of the day, and when it comes to the circadian diet, it holds true. A nourishing breakfast sets the tone for the rest of your day, providing you with sustained energy and essential nutrients. Let's explore some energizing breakfast options that will kick-start your morning.

Sunrise Smoothie Bowl:

Blend together a frozen banana, a handful of spinach, a scoop of protein powder, a tablespoon of almond butter, and a splash of almond milk. Top with fresh berries, sliced almonds, and a sprinkle of chia seeds. This vibrant smoothie bowl is packed with vitamins, minerals, and healthy fats to fuel your day.

Veggie Omelet:

Whisk together eggs, diced bell peppers, spinach, and cherry tomatoes. Cook in a non-stick skillet with a drizzle of olive oil until the omelet is set. Serve with a side of whole-grain toast and sliced avocado for a balanced and satisfying breakfast.

Overnight Chia Pudding:

Combine chia seeds, almond milk, and a touch of honey or maple syrup in a jar. Stir well and refrigerate overnight. In the morning, top with your favorite fruits, nuts, and a sprinkle of cinnamon for a delicious and nutrient-packed breakfast.

4.2 Satisfying Lunch Ideas:

Lunchtime is an opportunity to refuel your body and nourish yourself with a well-rounded meal. Let's explore some satisfying lunch ideas that will keep you energized throughout the day.

Quinoa Salad:

Toss cooked quinoa with a variety of colorful vegetables such as cucumbers, cherry tomatoes, bell peppers, and chopped herbs. Add a protein source like grilled chicken, chickpeas, or tofu. Drizzle with a homemade vinaigrette made from olive oil, lemon juice, and Dijon mustard for a refreshing and nutritious lunch.

Lentil Soup:

Simmer lentils, diced carrots, celery, onions, and garlic in a vegetable broth until tender. Season with herbs and spices like cumin, turmeric, and paprika for added flavor and health benefits. This hearty and fiber-rich soup will keep you satisfied and nourished.

Salmon Salad Wrap: Flake cooked salmon and mix it with Greek yogurt, lemon juice, diced cucumbers, and fresh dill. Spread the mixture onto a whole-grain wrap, add a handful of baby spinach, and roll it up for a protein-packed and portable lunch option.

4.3 Wholesome Dinner Delights:

Dinnertime is a time to unwind and enjoy a nourishing meal that supports your circadian health. Let's explore some wholesome dinner options that will satisfy your taste buds and provide essential nutrients.

Baked Chicken with Roasted Vegetables: Season chicken breasts with herbs and spices of your choice, such as rosemary, thyme, and garlic powder. Place the chicken on a baking sheet along with a medley of colorful vegetables like Brussels sprouts, carrots, and sweet potatoes. Drizzle with olive oil and bake until the chicken is cooked through and the vegetables are tender. This flavorful and balanced meal will delight your palate and provide a boost of protein and fiber.

Stir-Fried Tofu and Vegetables:

Sauté tofu cubes with a variety of sliced vegetables, such as bell peppers, broccoli, and snap peas. Add a splash of low-sodium soy sauce, minced ginger, and garlic for flavor. Serve over a bed of brown rice or quinoa for a satisfying and plant-based dinner option.

Grilled Shrimp Skewers with Quinoa Pilaf:

Thread marinated shrimp onto skewers and grill until cooked. Prepare a quinoa pilaf by sautéing diced onions, garlic, and mixed vegetables. Add cooked quinoa, vegetable broth, and herbs like parsley and lemon zest. Serve the grilled shrimp skewers over the quinoa pilaf for a light and flavorful dinner.

4.4 Snacks and Desserts:

Snacks and desserts can be enjoyed as part of the circadian diet while keeping the focus on nutrient-dense ingredients. Here are some ideas to satisfy your cravings.

Apple Slices with Almond Butter:

Slice crisp apple wedges and serve with a dollop of almond butter. The combination of sweet and savory flavors provides a satisfying and nutrient-packed snack.

Yogurt Parfait:

Layer Greek yogurt with fresh berries, granola, and a drizzle of honey. This parfait is not only delicious but also rich in protein, fiber, and antioxidants.

Dark Chocolate Energy Bites: Combine dates, nuts, cocoa powder, and a touch of honey in a food processor. Roll the mixture into small balls and refrigerate. These indulgent energy bites provide a healthy dose of antioxidants and natural sweetness.

Conclusion: Congratulations! You have now discovered a treasure trove of nourishing meal ideas and recipes that align with the principles of the circadian diet. From energizing breakfast options to satisfying lunches, wholesome dinners, and delightful snacks and desserts, you have a plethora of choices to support your circadian health and well-being.

Remember to embrace variety, experiment with flavors, and listen to your body's cues for hunger and satiety. Enjoy the process of nourishing yourself with vibrant and nutrient-dense foods, and let the circadian diet transform not only your plate but your overall vitality and quality of life.

In the next chapter, we will delve into the science behind the circadian diet, exploring its impact on various aspects of health, including weight management, metabolism, and longevity. So get ready to deepen your understanding of the remarkable benefits of the circadian diet and unlock its full potential.

Everything to Know About Your Circadian Rhythm

Your circadian rhythm helps control your daily schedule for sleep and wakefulness. This rhythm is tied to your 24-hour body clock, and most living things have one. Your circadian rhythm is influenced by outside things like light and dark, as well as other factors. Your brain receives signals based on your environment and activates certain hormones, alters your body temperature, and regulates your metabolism to keep you alert or draw you to sleep.

Some may experience disruptions to their circadian rhythm because of external factors or sleep disorders. Maintaining healthy habits can help you respond better to this natural rhythm of your body.

How it works

There are several components that make up your body's circadian rhythm. It is one of four biological rhythms in the body.

Cells in your body

First, cells in your brain respond to light and dark. Your eyes capture such changes in the environment and then send signals to different cells about when it's time to be sleepy or awake.

Those cells then send more signals to other parts of the brain that activate other functions that make you more tired or alert.

Hormones play a role

Hormones like melatonin and cortisol may increase or decrease as part of your circadian rhythm. Melatonin is a hormone that makes you sleepy, and your body releases more of it at night and suppresses it during the day. Cortisol can make you more alert, and your body produces more of it in the morning.

Other factors

Body temperature and metabolism are also part of your circadian rhythm. Your temperature drops when you sleep and rises during awake hours. Additionally, your metabolism works at different rates throughout the day.

Other factors may also influence your circadian rhythm. Your rhythm may adjust based on your work hours, physical activity, and additional habits or lifestyle choices.

Age is another factor that influences your circadian rhythm. Infants, teens, and adults all experience circadian rhythms differently.

Circadian rhythm in babies

Newborns do not have a circadian rhythm developed until they are a few months old. This can cause their sleeping patterns to be erratic in the first days, weeks, and months of their lives. Their circadian rhythm develops as they adapt to the environment and experience changes to their bodies. Babies begin to release melatonin when they are about three months old, and the hormone cortisol develops from 2 months to 9 months old.

Toddlers and children have a fairly regulated sleep schedule once their circadian rhythm and corresponding body functions mature. Children need about 9 or 10 hours of sleep a night.

Circadian rhythm in teens

Teenagers experience a shift in their circadian rhythm known as sleep phase delay. Unlike in their childhood years with early bedtimes around 8 or 9 p.m., teenagers may not get tired until much later in the night.

Melatonin may not rise until closer to 10 or 11 p.m. or even later. That shift also results in a teenager's need to sleep later in the morning. Their peak sleepy hours at night are from 3 a.m. to 7 a.m. — or may even be later —

but they still need the same amount of sleep as children.

Circadian rhythm in adults

Adults should have a pretty consistent circadian rhythm if they practice healthy habits. Their bedtimes and wake times should remain stable if they follow a fairly regular schedule and aim for seven to nine hours of sleep every night. Adults likely get sleepy well before midnight, as melatonin releases into their bodies. They reach their most tired phases of the day from 2 to 4 a.m. and 1 to 3 p.m.

Older adults may notice their circadian rhythm changes with age, and they begin to go to bed earlier than they used to and wake in the wee hours of the morning. In general, this is a normal part of aging.

How it gets out of sync

Sometimes it is not possible to follow your circadian rhythm, and your lifestyle needs and internal clock clash. This can occur because of:

- Overnight or off-hours work shifts that go against the natural light and dark times of day.

- Work shifts with erratic hours.

- Travel that spans the course of one or more different time zones.

- A lifestyle that encourages late-night hours or early wake times.

- Medications you take.

- Stress.

- Mental health conditions.

- Health conditions like brain damage, dementia, head injuries, or blindness.

• Poor sleep habits, including lacking a sleep schedule, eating, or drinking late at night, watching screens too close to bedtime, or not having a comfortable sleeping space.

How to reset

You may experience disruptions to your circadian rhythm, but you can get it back on track. Here are some tips for promoting a healthy 24-hour schedule:

• Try to adhere to a routine each day.

• Spend time outdoors when it's light outside to boost your wakefulness.

- Get enough daily exercise — twenty or more minutes of aerobic exercise is generally recommended.

- Sleep in an environment that promotes rest with proper lighting, a comfortable temperature, and a supportive mattress.

- Avoid alcohol, caffeine, and nicotine in the evenings.

- Power down your screens well before bedtime and try engaging in something analog, such as reading a book or meditating.

• Do not nap late in the afternoon or evening.

Sleep disorders

Sometimes alterations to your circadian rhythm may be the sign of a more serious condition like a circadian rhythm sleep disorder. Two of these disorders are advanced sleep phase and delayed sleep phase. You may be more susceptible to these if you work an irregular shift, are blind, or are a teenager or older adult.

Delayed sleep phase disorder occurs when you go to bed and awaken two hours or more after most people. You may think of yourself as a "night owl." Teenagers and young adults are more prone to this condition.

Advanced sleep phase disorder is the opposite of delayed sleep phase disorder. You actually fall asleep a few hours before most people and then awaken very early in the morning.

Disorders related to your circadian rhythm may result in having difficulty falling asleep at night, waking frequently throughout the night, and waking and not being able to go back to sleep in the middle of the night.

Symptoms related to these conditions include:

- insomnia

- sleep loss

- problems waking in the morning

- tiredness throughout the day

- depression or stress

Other conditions that are tied into your circadian rhythm include:

- jet lag, caused from traveling over several time zones quickly

- shift work disorder, caused by an off-hours job or a job with unpredictable hours

- irregular sleep-wake disorder, caused by an inability to set a regular sleep and wake schedule

Treating these conditions may include a variety of approaches. You may try to:

- set a more regular schedule

- use light therapy

- take medications or supplements like melatonin to fall asleep more easily

- try an intentional shift in your sleep implemented over several days or weeks

Health effects

Maintaining your circadian rhythm is vital to your health. If you experience a disruption to your circadian rhythm and struggle to get the proper amount of sleep, you may experience both short-term and long-term consequences to your health.

Disruption to your circadian rhythm can cause health conditions in several parts of the body in the long term. This includes your:

- organs

- cardiovascular system

- metabolism

- gastrointestinal system

- skin

You may be more susceptible to diabetes, obesity, and mental health conditions as well.

Short-term disruptions to your circadian rhythm may result in problems with memory or lack of energy. It may also take longer to heal an injury if you don't get enough sleep.

When to talk with a doctor

There are several reasons you may want to talk to a doctor about an issue with your circadian rhythm. If you experience one of these issues for a prolonged period, consider making a doctor's appointment:

• Have trouble achieving adequate sleep every night

- Cannot fall asleep easily

- Awaken several times a night and fail to get quality sleep

- Have trouble waking up

- Feel extremely tired during waking hours

The bottom line

Your circadian rhythm is your body's natural way of keeping to its 24-hour body clock, helping your body operate on a healthy sleep-wake schedule. Living a healthy, active lifestyle that promotes proper rest will help you maintain this important component of your body.

Reach out to your doctor if you experience prolonged difficulties sleeping or extreme fatigue during the day to find out how you can realign with your circadian rhythm and get proper rest.

The Effects of Sleep Deprivation on Your Body

If you've ever spent a night tossing and turning, you already know how you'll feel the next day — tired, cranky, and out of sorts. But missing out on the recommended 7 to 9 hours of shut-eye nightly does more than make you feel groggy and grumpy.

The long-term effects of sleep deprivation are real.

It drains your mental abilities and puts your physical health at real risk. Science has linked poor slumber with a number of health problems, from weight gain to a weakened immune system.

Read on to learn the causes of sleep deprivation and exactly how it affects specific body functions and systems.

Causes of sleep deprivation

In a nutshell, sleep deprivation is caused by consistent lack of sleep or reduced quality of sleep. Getting less than 7 hours of sleep on a regular basis can eventually lead to health consequences that affect your entire body. This may also be caused by an underlying sleep disorder.

Your body needs sleep, just as it needs air and food to function at its best.

During sleep, your body heals itself and restores its chemical balance. Your brain forges new thought connections and helps memory retention.

Without enough sleep, your brain and body systems won't function normally. It can also dramatically lower your quality of life.

A review of studies in 2010Trusted Source found that sleeping too little at night increases the risk of early death.

Noticeable signs of sleep deprivation include:

- excessive sleepiness

- frequent yawning

- irritability

- daytime fatigue

Stimulants, such as caffeine, aren't enough to override your body's profound need for sleep. In fact, these can make sleep deprivation worse by making it harder to fall asleep at night.

This, in turn, may lead to a cycle of nighttime insomnia followed by daytime caffeine consumption to combat the tiredness caused by the lost hours of shut-eye.

Behind the scenes, chronic sleep deprivation can interfere with your body's internal systems and cause more than just the initial signs and symptoms listed above.

Central nervous system

Your central nervous system is the main information highway of your body. Sleep is necessary to keep it functioning properly, but chronic insomnia can disrupt how your body usually sends and processes information.

During sleep, pathways form between nerve cells (neurons) in your brain that help you remember new information you've learned. Sleep deprivation leaves your brain exhausted, so it can't perform its duties as well.

You may also find it more difficult to concentrate or learn new things. The signals your body sends may also be delayed, decreasing your coordination and increasing your risk for accidents.

Sleep deprivation also negatively affects your mental abilities and emotional state. You may feel more impatient or prone to mood swings. It can also compromise decision-making processes and creativity.

If sleep deprivation continues long enough, you could start having hallucinations — seeing or hearing things that aren't really there. A lack of sleep can also trigger mania in people who have bipolar mood disorder. Other psychological risks include:

• impulsive behavior

• anxiety

• depression

- paranoia

- suicidal thoughts

You may also end up experiencing microsleep during the day. During these episodes, you'll fall asleep for a few to several seconds without realizing it.

Microsleep is out of your control and can be extremely dangerous if you're driving. It can also make you more prone to injury if you operate heavy machinery at work and have a microsleep episode.

Immune system

While you sleep, your immune system produces protective, infection-fighting substances like antibodies and cytokines. It uses these substances to combat foreign invaders such as bacteria and viruses.

Certain cytokines also help you to sleep, giving your immune system more efficiency to defend your body against illness.

Sleep deprivation prevents your immune system from building up its forces. If you don't get enough sleep, your body may not be able to fend off invaders, and it may also take you longer to recover from illness.

Long-term sleep deprivation also increases your risk for chronic conditions, such as diabetes mellitus and heart disease.

Respiratory system

The relationship between sleep and the respiratory system goes both ways. A nighttime breathing disorder called obstructive sleep apnea (OSA) can interrupt your sleep and lower sleep quality.

As you wake up throughout the night, this can cause sleep deprivation, which leaves you more vulnerable to respiratory infections like the common cold and flu. Sleep deprivation can also make existing respiratory diseases worse, such as chronic lung illness.

Digestive system

Along with eating too much and not exercising, sleep deprivation is another risk factor for becoming overweight and obese. Sleep affects the levels of two hormones, leptin and ghrelin, which control feelings of hunger and fullness.

Leptin tells your brain that you've had enough to eat. Without enough sleep, your brain reduces leptin and raises ghrelin, which is an appetite stimulant. The flux of these hormones could explain nighttime snacking or why someone may overeat later in the night.

A lack of sleep can also make you feel too tired to exercise. Over time, reduced physical activity can make you gain weight because you're not burning enough calories and not building muscle mass.

Sleep deprivation also causes your body to release less insulin after you eat. Insulin helps to reduce your blood sugar (glucose) level.

Sleep deprivation also lowers the body's tolerance for glucose and is associated with insulin resistance. These disruptions can lead to diabetes mellitus and obesity.

Cardiovascular system

Sleep affects processes that keep your heart and blood vessels healthy, including those that affect your blood sugar, blood pressure, and inflammation levels. It also plays a vital role in your body's ability to heal and repair the blood vessels and heart.

People who don't sleep enough are more likely to get cardiovascular disease. One analysis linked insomnia to an increased risk of heart attack and stroke.

Endocrine system

Hormone production is dependent on your sleep. For testosterone production, you need at least 3 hours of uninterrupted sleep, which is about the time of your first R.E.M. episode. Waking up throughout the night could affect hormone production.

This interruption can also affect growth hormone production, especially in children and adolescents. These hormones help the body build muscle mass and repair cells and tissues, in addition to other growth functions.

The pituitary gland releases growth hormone throughout each day, but adequate sleep and exercise also help the release of this hormone.

Treatment for sleep deprivation

The most basic form of sleep deprivation treatment is getting an adequate amount of sleep, typically 7 to 9 hours each night.

This is often easier said than done, especially if you've been deprived of precious shut-eye for several weeks or longer. After this point, you may need help from your doctor or a sleep specialist who, if needed, can diagnose and treat a possible sleep disorder.

Sleep disorders may make it difficult to get quality sleep at night. They may also increase your risk for the above effects of sleep deprivation on the body.

The following are some of the most common types of sleep disorders:

- obstructive sleep apnea

- narcolepsy

- restless leg syndrome

- insomnia

- circadian rhythm disorders

To diagnose these conditions, your doctor may order a sleep study. This is traditionally conducted at a formal sleep center, but now there are options to measure your sleep quality at home, too.

If you're diagnosed with a sleep disorder, you may be given medication or a device to keep your airway open at night (in the case of obstructive sleep apnea) to help combat the disorder so you can get a better night's sleep on a regular basis.

Prevention

The best way to prevent sleep deprivation is to make sure you get adequate sleep. Follow the recommended guidelines for your age group, which is 7 to 9 hours for most adults ages 18 to 64.

Other ways you can get back on track with a healthy sleep schedule include:

- limiting daytime naps (or avoiding them altogether)

- refraining from caffeine past noon or at least a few hours prior to bedtime

- going to bed at the same time each night

- waking up at the same time every morning

- sticking to your bedtime schedule during weekends and holidays

- spending an hour before bed doing relaxing activities, such as reading, meditating, or taking a bath

- avoiding heavy meals within a few hours before bedtime

- refraining from using electronic devices right before bed

- exercising regularly, but not in the evening hours close to bedtime

- reducing alcohol intake

If you continue to have problems sleeping at night and are fighting daytime fatigue, talk to your doctor. They can test for underlying health conditions that might be getting in the way of your sleep schedule.

Printed in Great Britain
by Amazon

26773494R00056